Psychosis and the Humpty-Dumpty Story

Curtis L.V. Adams MD

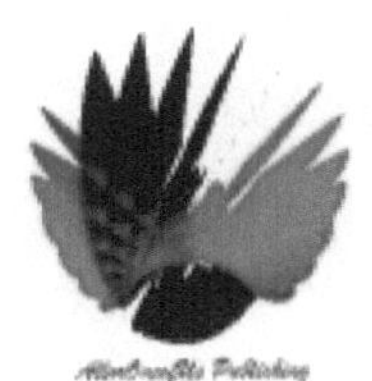

AllrOneofUs Publishing
Baltimore, Md & Huntsville, Al

While every precaution has been taken in the preparation of this book, the publisher assumes no responsibility for errors or omissions, or for damages resulting from the use of the information contained herein.

PSYCHOSIS AND THE HUMPTY-DUMPTY STORY

First edition. June 18, 2020.

ISBN: 978-1393016496

Written by Curtis L.V. Adams, M.D..

Table of Contents

FOREWARD 1
PREFACE AND BRIEF BIOGRAPHY BY DR. CURTIS ADAMS 3
INTRODUCTION: MY PERSONAL DEVELOPMENT 5
CHAPTER I: PSYCHOSIS AND THE HUMPTY DUMPTY STORY 13
CHAPTER II: TREATMENT IMPLICATIONS OF VARIOUS ATTITUDES TOWARDS MENTAL ILLNESS 25
CHAPTER III: DEPRESSION 31
CHAPTER IV: BIOLOGY OF RELATIONAL SYSTEMS 39
CHAPTER VI: AIKIDO AND MIND-BODY INTEGRATION 47
APPENDIX: MEDITATION 57
BIBLIOGRAPHY 59

This work is dedicated to the patients who have been willing to stay with me until the resolution of their problems. When one middle-aged lady came in with her son acting out, I got him straightened out and worked through the lady's feelings about her own mother after she ended a poor marriage. She went on to take a promotion in Washington. At her last session, she came in with a quote from a book on Zen that I had given her. The Zen student in the book said, "I curse the day I heard the word Zen, but I would take nothing for the benefit it has been for me." Then she said, "I have cursed the day I heard the name Dr. Adams, but I would take nothing for the benefit he has been for me."

FOREWARD

An event in space-time some 45 years ago joined my life, when I had just started college, with that of a young psychiatrist who was beginning his practice in the deep south. He helped guide me through a symbolic process which was at the time diagnosed as a "reactive manic-depressive episode." Instead of drugging and dampening down the symptoms, the psychiatrist allowed the process, listening carefully and helping to guide the symptoms into some structure. As the Jungian John Weir Perry has said, he was making a "container" for the experience. It was an experience which Dr. Adams described at the time as a "creative burst."

It's important to note that real pain and suffering accompany such experiences, which evoke classic symptoms of "end of the world," polarization of good and evil, and seeing the world through a symbolic lens. Those elements were present, but the ability to pass through the experience made all the difference, and Dr. Adams helped make that possible. This was back in the days when there was still psychoanalytic understanding and practices such as "kind firmness."

I was one of his early patients, but Curtis Adams went on to work in the field for decades, helping many other patients. It is time to listen to these writings, some of which have their origins years ago and others more recently. They show a path that points us toward true healing in mental health.

Michael Susko, Editor

PREFACE AND BRIEF BIOGRAPHY BY DR. CURTIS ADAMS

I was born in 1934 at the height of the Great Depression as the first child to a share-cropper family and grew up in abject poverty. My father could neither read nor write but valued education and insured that his four children attended school. From an early age, I wanted to become a physician and was helped towards that goal by my teachers. I was able to go get a college degree and one year of medical school on the G.I. Bill. Borrowing money was easy after that.

After four years in general practice, I gave in to my love for psychiatry and went back to school to become a psychiatrist. Growing up had prepared me for that, and my years in general practice sealed the deal. I went to the Philadelphia Child Guidance Clinic to learn about families and to study with Jay Haley. During my training, I began my studies in alternative views of the psychotic process and how to treat the person undergoing such a process. Haley's book *Strategies of Psychotherapy* was one of the most important books in my development.

I practiced psychiatry for 45 years before retiring. The papers in this collection are the result of continued study as questions arose around patients in my practice. I think that a psychiatrist has to be able to fit into the prevailing view of mental illness, and I have not been able to make that fit.

INTRODUCTION: MY PERSONAL DEVELOPMENT

Michael Susko referred to my unpublished paper "Psychosis and the Humpty-Dumpty Story" in his paper "Caseness and Narrative" published in *The Journal of Mind and Behavior*. He has urged me to publish the paper for some time and has found a way we can publish the paper along with some related lectures and papers I have written over my 45 years as a psychiatrist, along with this introduction.

When I quit my residency in ophthalmology to enter psychiatry, my mentor Marie DuBalen, a French nurse turned social worker, sent me the French proverb, "If you chase away the obvious, it will come back on a galloping horse."

Given my family history and experiences growing up, summarized here and to be expanded in a future work, my destiny to become a psychiatrist should have been obvious to me.

I was the oldest child and grandchild born into a family of sharecroppers. My mother was ambitious and thought she was marrying up because my grandfather had a store, which he maintained to supply needs of the sharecroppers on the farm for which he was the overseer. My father had walked some twenty miles each way to see her on weekends. Apparently, she realized her mistake quickly after they married.

My father, eldest of thirteen children, attended school only a few days in first and second grades. He could neither read nor write. In addition to plowing cotton fields at age six, he and his oldest sister were surrogate parents for the other ten children, as their mother was severely hypochondriacal until her death. He grew up to be regarded as a "good man and a good worker."

He was always acutely aware of his lack of education and taught his four children that, "If you get an education, nobody can take it away from you." My older sister and I tried to teach him to read and to do simple arithmetic so that he could qualify for a promotion where he worked. He would manifest such severe frustration that we all gave up on the project. I think he had an organic learning disorder. An uncle told me that he himself "had earned to read several times, but it had leaked out." Of my dad's four children, there is an M.D., a Ph.D., a social worker, and a government computer specialist. We got the message.

I remember growing up as a time of fear, manifest by extreme leg pains, which my father treated at night with Sloan's Liniment and leg rubs. I later learned that my mother beat me to the point that my dad thought she would kill me. Rage reactions from my uncles, just a little older than me, also contributed to my chronic fear. Later that fear was sometimes manifested in my untimely rages, which accompanied me through early adult life. I considered the rages as uncontrolled anger. Now I know them to be fear, as in "the cornered rat state." By the seventh grade, I had learned to fight and was the protector of the other "brains", so I was less afraid.

In a therapy session, I asked my therapist why, after my "successes", all the growing up hardships were important. He said, "They leave scars." Quite an understatement. He did not say the scars extend to the cellular level, as did Georg Groddeck in the *Book of the It* or that they interfere with essential energy flow in the body as did Wilhelm Reich in *The Function of the Orgone*. Perhaps he did not know, or those bits of data were not part of the dogma of his sect. I learned how limiting sectarian dogma can be during my three years as a minister in a Christian Sect.

When about four, I had an experience of wonderful clarity, which I have had described to me by only one patient. That was on a day when my mother was in a good mood, had baked doughnuts and allowed me to sit on the back steps of our shack to eat the doughnuts. The day was clear with a warm breeze. The feeling lasted for what seemed like a long time. I think the feeling is that called *Joy* by Nina Bull.

I selected medicine as a career when I was in my second year of first grade and had a discussion of jobs with one of my uncles. He thought being a physician was better than being a lawyer, which my mother recommended. The reason being money. Whatever the motivation, that was always my stated goal. After I became a straight A student in the fourth grade, my teachers pointed me toward my stated goal. After I was older, I compared what I learned about other jobs and professions to what I was learning about medicine and stayed on that track. Perhaps my father's migraines, my mother's smothering spells, and my intensely psychosomatic grandmother helped.

I maintained a state of fear-of-poverty, failure, and interpersonal relationships for many years. My rages did not get me into too much trouble and prevented bullying. I identified the emotion fear and learned what I now sometimes tell patients, "Feel the fear, and do it anyway."

Psychiatry was the only subject taught for all four years of medical school in my time. I developed my abhorrence for ECT there. I also developed my interest in mind-body relationships during the weekly conference on psychosomatic medicine during my senior year. I had a two-month part time assignment in psychiatry during my internship.

I then went into general practice and emergency room work, both of which convinced me of the truth in the statement that at least sixty percent of visits to physicians are for psychiatric (psychosomatic?) reasons. I also learned during that time that simple counseling helped many of the patients through those complaints. They did not want a pill, as many of my colleagues argued, but help with their problems.

By the time I began my psychiatric residency, I had read many of the books we were required to read and had seen most of the conditions presenting in the psychiatric setting. I had also learned of the lack of success from treatment with antianxiety medications and the brain damage done by electroshock treatment, the psychiatric cash cow. I was ready to learn something better.

During residency I had a modified "training analysis" which helped me to begin the process of looking at my own "issues" and to be more open to seeing the effect of poor parenting, poverty, extended family, etc. on my own life and the lives of my patients.

Jay Haley's *Strategies of Psychotherapy* gave me my first insight into the different levels of the systems surrounding the development of a psychiatric problem and the thinking necessary to establish a therapeutic relationship with the patient. I also began to see the mental breakdown as a result of treatment of the patient by family, school, and other social systems in which he lived. I did not know about the limbic system yet and had not coined the phrase "limbic system failure."

My brother, after hearing me express my problems reconciling the various systems of psychology, introduced me to General Semantics, the epistemological system of Alfred Korzybski. Intense study of writings of that group helped me to resolve many of the contradictions by understanding the level of abstraction involved in the conclusions of the various pilgrims in the mental health field. It was at a General Semantics seminar that I experienced my first episode of heightened sense of awareness.

Betty Keene led the group in what they called "Sensory Awareness." Afterwards, I got off the floor and sat in a chair. I did not know I could feel so tired. Through a week of lectures and awareness and other exercises, I discovered what Trigant Burrow describes as the difference between self-objectivation and self-awareness. This was the beginning of my journey towards healing. Suffice it to say that people in the Psychiatry Department did not see the change as growth, but as mental illness. They were kind enough to protect me or maybe better themselves and allow me to finish my second year there. That was when I began to see the attitude towards mental illness.

My first "reactive psychotic episode" was at the same time thrilling and alarming. I was not in my familiar protected state, nor in complete control. Over the years, I have had the attitude towards my experience as I see in most "recovering people"—Guilt (fear I will be punished by loss of status) and shame (fear I will lose the positive regard of others).

Trigant Burrow thought one could shift his attitude by focusing on feelings around his eyes. He did not call his work meditation, but I learned that fixing one's eyes (stopping saccadic motion of the eyes) is central to all meditation. I continued that study through General Semantics workshops, Zen, and Aikido. My instruction paper on the essentials of meditation is enclosed. It is one way to continue to process stored information about our history and resolve the attitudes and thoughts derived from our traumas, i.e. complete the psychotic process, heal the wounds.

During my child psychiatry fellowship, I watched one of the other Fellows treat a family with a child diagnosed with schizophrenia. As the therapist ignored the child and worked with the parents on their marriage and communication, the child stopped acting as if he was talking to someone else in the room and joined the parents and therapist. He joined in the family discussion and showed no abnormality in the future sessions that I watched through the one-way mirror. My own cases there, under the supervision of people not wed to the idea of mental illness, improved my skills. However, when I presented a case of a young boy referred with the diagnosis and no longer showing symptoms after treatment, I was told, "If you cured him, he was not autistic." Both cases belie the permeance of psychiatric conditions.

At the end of my first year of Child Psychiatry, I was eligible to take my General Psychiatry Boards, so I was in that state of letting my guard down and not being so subservient. At the same time, I participated in a therapy intensive. I lapsed into a psychotic state resulting in a psychiatric hospitalization. Luckily for me, my psychiatrist was a master therapist, and allowed me to continue in my process, supporting and advising me. The Director of the Clinic and the Training Director visited me in the hospital and decided I could come back after I was able to concentrate on work. I continued working on the process for some time. Aikido was a great help, and I continued my exercise and meditation.

In my first few years in practice, I had a clinic with several other therapists. We called it The Institute for Personal Change. Several of my papers were the outgrowth of our work together. I also taught medical students during that time, which was a stimulus to study. It was during that time that we explored the concept of the "Creative Illness" as in the enclosed paper. Jung and his Bollingen Tower series are my favorite examples of the work and support the psychotic process requires. Had Jung known about the third division of the limbic system, his presentation of the importance of symbols might have been different.

Growth groups called "T" groups were popular during the early 1970s. During that time, I saw several people with what we called then "brief reactive psychoses". Those cases gave "T" groups a bad name but provided me with new experience and supported the view that psychosis is not all bad. The patients had new insights into their lives and were able to reconstitute quickly. I also saw psychosis induced by nitrous oxide and marijuana. Some of those people were interested enough and disturbed enough to continue with me until we agreed they were to the normal end of the process.

The papers included in this collection were written over a long period, and hopefully complement each other. Study of the limbic system of the brain provides insight into the organic nature of emotions. The Attitudinal Theory of Emotions, along with the limbic system, provides a basis for understanding depression.

I am working on a more unified book, which I hope to complete soon.

CHAPTER I: PSYCHOSIS AND THE HUMPTY DUMPTY STORY

A quote: "It would appear that once precipitated into psychosis, the patient has a course to run. He is, as it were, embarked upon a voyage of discovery which is only completed by his return to the normal world to which he comes back with insights different from those of the inhabitants who never embarked upon such a voyage. Once begun, a schizophrenic episode would appear to have as definite a course as an initiation ceremony-a death and re-birth-into which the novice may have been precipitated by his family life or by adventitious circumstance, but which in its course is largely steered by an endogenous process.

In terms of this picture, spontaneous remission is no problem. This is only the final and natural outcome of the total process. What needs to be explained is the failure of many who embark upon this voyage to return from it. Do these encounter circumstances either in family life or in institutional care so grossly maladaptive that even the richest and best organized hallucinatory experience cannot save them?"

The quote is from Gregory Bateson's preface to *Percival's Narrative: A Patient's Account of His Psychosis, 1830-1832*. My premise is that the answer to the question posed is, "Yes, they do". They encounter circumstances either in family life or in institutional care so grossly maladaptive that even the richest and best organized hallucinatory experience cannot save them. Very often, the problem is in the institutional care patients receive. The responsibility we have when we admit someone to a psychiatric hospital or unit is to make sure that what we do does not prevent the natural outcome of the "psychotic" experience.

Since I believe that the "psychotic" process has a natural, predictable course that must be carried through, it seems necessary to explain how the process starts and what it means in terms of the human experience.

From here on, I will use the term "psychosis" to mean nervous break-down and to apply to the neurotic states and the psychosomatic conditions as well as to schizophrenia and the functional manic states. The logic of this usage will become apparent as I proceed.

It is generally agreed by all schools of thought that development proceeds in a stage-wise manner. There is an organic process which has to do with growth of the body.

There are certain things a person learns to do regardless of what happens to his personality. People learn to eat, digest their food, eliminate, to move about, etc. This process represents the organic component of development. However, there is a mental component of development, a development of the personality, which proceeds stage-wise, starting with the oral stage. The patient accrues enough mental schema to deal with oral activities, and he develops a view of himself in the world, a mental "self" based on oral percepts. At the end of the oral stage, usually around twelve to fourteen months, there is a period of turmoil. During this process, the person's view of himself disorganizes, and he reorganizes his self-concept to be more nearly representative of the actual facts of himself and of the world. Part of the turmoil comes about when he realizes that he is not really omnipotent and he has to come back to his body to discover his limitations. There follows another period of accumulation of mental schema that we speak of as the anal stage; then there is another disorganization phase, during which time the patient again brings his world view back into touch with his body. Then follows the phallic stage, etc. (See Figure 1).

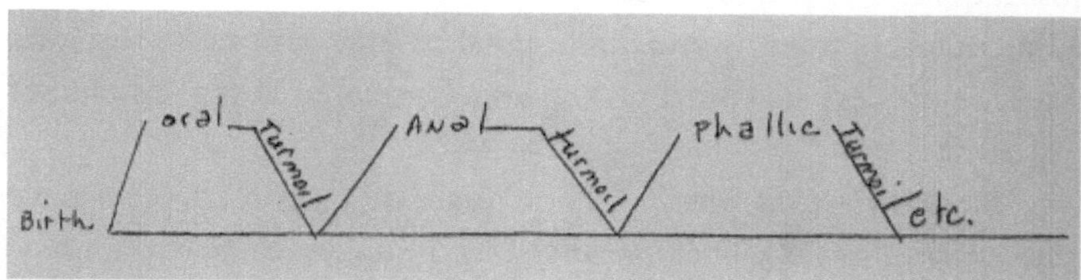

Figure 1

Development is a process of accumulating mental data which is often not in touch with reality. In other words, there is a self-representation and self-world representation that is objectified, schematized, etc., that does not always correspond to the facts of the person, nor to himself in the world. The person has to undergo a disorganization of these objectifications and schematizations, sift through the mental data, and bring his images back into touch with the reality of the limitations of his own body, abilities and powers, and to the limitations and boundaries imposed by the world. This process, when it is not interfered with, proceeds naturally and automatically.

There is a disorganization period at the end of each of the stages of development. The disorganization-reorganization process can be completed only if it is supported by the environment. If the environment punishes or interferes with the process, the person will maintain his view of himself and of the world, based upon information and mis-information which he has accrued during the previous stage. The accrual of mis-information can be cumulative from more than one previous stage.

The primary element of the environment for support of the development process is the family. In order for the family to function properly, it must receive support from the larger society. It is my belief that practically no family, and practically no structured environmental social system, allows or supports a disorganization phase. As a result, "everyone", with a very few possible exceptions, develops abnormally. We have the situation in which there is gradually increasing separation between the objectified, conceptualized view of the world and the self, and the real person. Practically everyone carries with him some omnipotence that goes with the oral stage; some fear, frugality, etc., that goes with the anal stage; some desire to control, etc., that goes with the phallic stage of development; practically everyone is either afraid of, or hates, his parents; and practically no one knows where he fits into the real world.

The result of this lack of permission and support of periodic developmental disorganization is a separation between the real self and what is called by Trigant Burrow, the "I-Persona". The latter is the self that most of us know, our social self, the self that we present to other people. It is what we say about ourselves. There is practically always a very wide split between the real self and the "I-Persona" (See Figure 2).

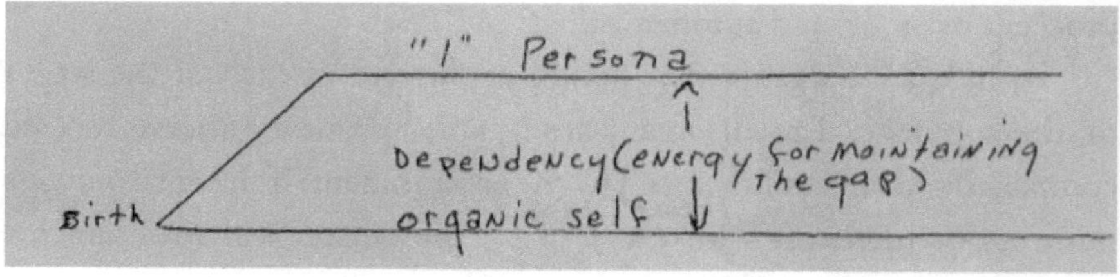

Figure 2

The "I-Persona" is that part of us which is validated by the environment. We are rewarded by the environment for living in a particular mode. Those upon whom we depend in our very early days help us to establish the definition of our false self. In a word, the force that maintains the split between the real self and the "I-Persona" is one's own dependency. If a person depends upon someone else, he acts in such a way as to please that person.

***

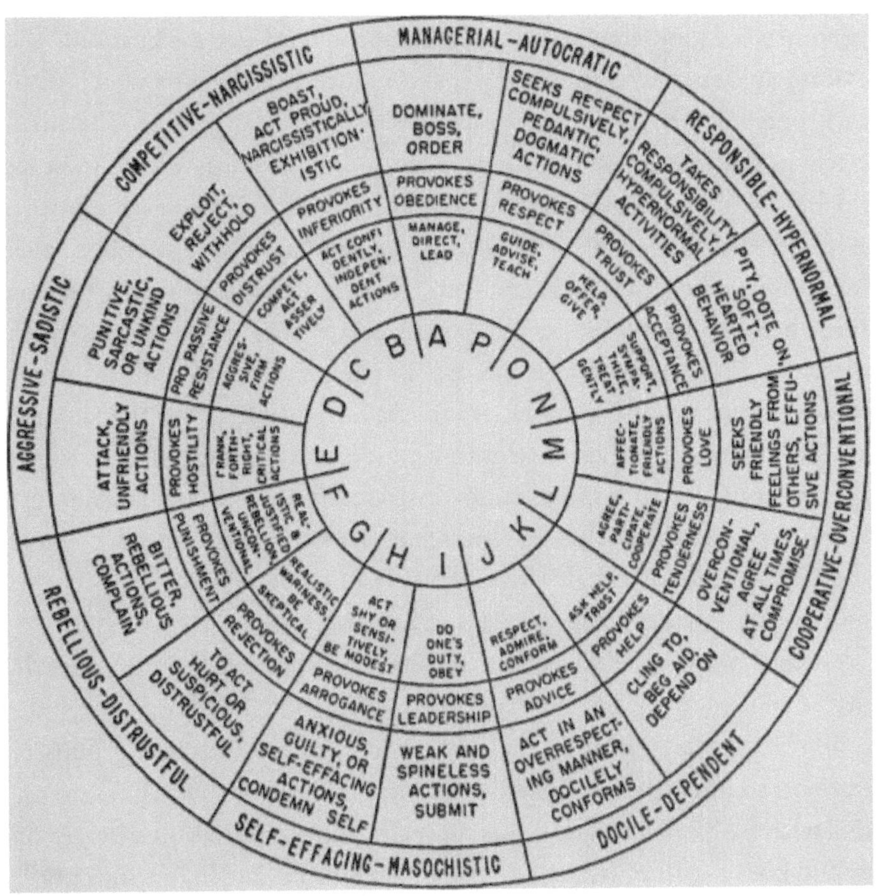

Figure 3

Figure 3 is reproduced from Timothy Leary's book, *Interpersonal Diagnosis of Personality*. It is a shortened version of Leary's attempt to systematize the "I-Persona" or the ways that people present themselves to other people in order to (1) alleviate their own anxiety, or (2) to get their dependency needs met. These may be actually the same motivator, stated in different terms.

The wheel is divided into eight different parts, with each part having an adaptive range and an extreme or maladaptive range. The small circle in the middle represents the adaptive range. The absolutely normal person would be able to use the behavior that fits a situation. The extremely character disordered person is stuck in behaviors which fit in only one segment of the wheel, usually in the extreme range. The small circle in the middle of the wheel is labeled with words which indicate the behavior which is elicited in groups by the behaviors in that segment. An often seen example is the Docile-Dependent woman we often label "depressed". She clings to, begs aid and depends on. She provokes helping from her environment. She has organized her internal schema in such a way that her "I-Persona" is that she is a helpless individual who needs to be taken care of by the environment. She has little, if any, anxiety and few, if any, psychiatric symptoms, except when she is unable to get the environment to respond in the expected way. When she fails to get her needs met, when her environment does not respond by helping, she intensifies her struggle to get the environment to help. She becomes more helpless, whiny, dependent, and begging.

Leary showed that as any person enters a group, he emits in increasing intensity his "interpersonal reflex" or "I-Persona" until the group responds to him in the way he has grown to expect groups to respond to him. He works harder and harder to make what he is doing, and what he has habitually done, succeed. If an aggressive, hostile person is put into a group, he will attack and be more and more unfriendly until the group responds with hostility. If a dependent person is placed into a group, he will become more and more dependent until the group responds to him by offering to help. Of course, if the person's behavior works, there is no reason to escalate the behavior or to give it up.

If the "I-Persona" does not work, the usual solution is to try harder to make it work. The person will invest more and more energy into his usual means of pleasing his environment, or into managing his own behavior. The energy available to the human organism is limited. One can produce only a certain number of ergs of energy during any given amount of time. A person can get into trouble by trying harder. The environment begins to react by rejecting the one-sided or one dimensional nature

of the person's behavior. We generally speak of that person as having a
personality disorder. (See Figure 4)

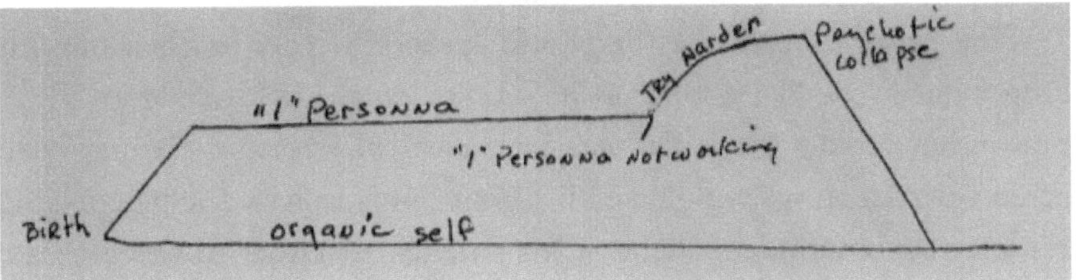

Figure 4

The usual outcome of the trying harder situation is that the personality
collapses (Figure 4). The Humpty-Dumpty nursery rhyme describes this
situation. Humpty Dumpty sat on a wall. Humpty-Dumpty had a great
fall. All the King's horses and all the King's men can't put the "I-Persona"
together again. Once it no longer works, it is not likely to ever work
again. People try, often, to reconstitute their "I-Personas", and clinicians
speak of a person's returning to his "premorbid personality"; however,
these attempts are usually not successful, and the "premorbid
personality" does not usually work after it has once decompensated.
Once a person begins to decompensate, he has only the choice of the
natural progression of the psychosis.

Suppose that one is a nurse whose job is to take care of others,
and she suddenly finds that people no longer want to be cared for. The
usually attempted solution is for her to try harder to care for them.
One day they will overtly reject her efforts to care, and then she is in
trouble. Suppose that one is a responsible, hyper-normal male married
to a docile, dependent woman. This is a frequently found combination.
If the docile, dependent woman decides that she no longer wants to be
docile, dependent, and that she wants to develop some independent life
of her own, the usual thing the man does is to try harder to manage
her life. If the man decides that he wants to change into a more open,

casual way of functioning, his docile, dependent wife usually escalates her dependent, helpless behavior until she finds herself being admitted to a hospital labeled as having an endogenous depression.

The other time that a "psychotic" process occurs is when one no longer needs the "I-Persona" as he has structured it (See Figure 5). A person has acted a particular way for a particular reason. He may have acted a particular way to please his parents, only to have the parents die. He may become independent of his parents. At either of those times, he may stop pouring energy into being the way the parents thought he should be.

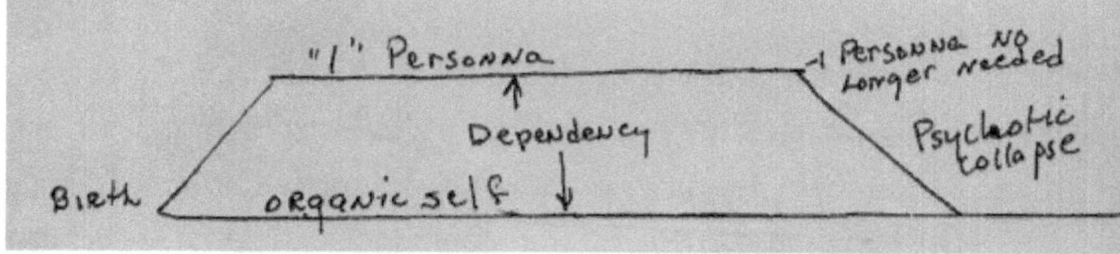

Figure 5

An example of this type of "psychosis" can be found in the offspring of members of a particular church of my acquaintance. These children leave home after having been reared in very protective environments. When they go away to college, 95% of them attend church only when they return home on vacations. Very often the "I-Persona" of the "good kid" disappears. They no longer pour energy into their "good kid" image as they have done when in the presence of and dependent upon their parents. The psychosis that appears in this situation is often diagnosed as schizophrenia or Dementia Praecox—that is, the craziness of the young. Once crazy, the only way is to complete the process. Shirley Jackson's *Hangsman* is a good fictional account of this process in a college freshman.

There is a predictable course in the psychotic process (See figure 6). The earliest symptoms are feelings. The usual psychiatric designation at this level is neurosis. The patient has intense anxiety, crying, or other manifestations of feeling disorders. The next level of symptoms is of thought disorders. Within this level is a layering out of the various kinds of thoughts described in Adlerian, Freudian, Rankian, and Jungian systems, respectively. Each of those systems describes different types of thinking processes. Adler described power struggles; Freud described struggles between mother, father, and child; Rank described birth and rebirth, being born again, being a new child; and Jungian psychology describes archetypes, such as the Christ archetype. There is a predictable ordering out in the psychotic process. After the thought disorders come the bodily reactions, generally seen as psychosomatic illnesses by family doctors.

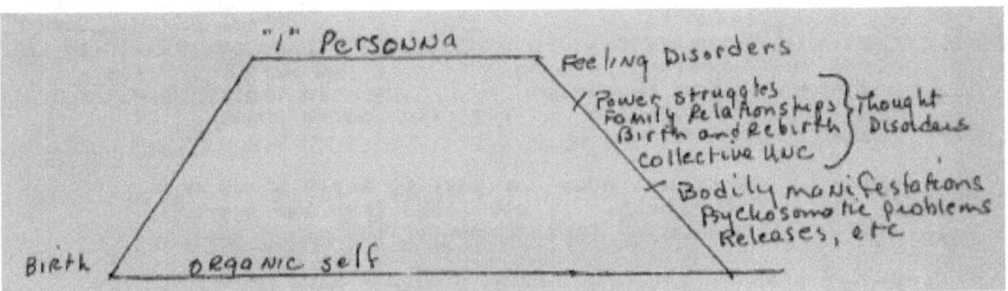

Figure 6

The job of the mental illness professional, then, is to see the person through the psychotic process. Once the person is finished with the process, his view of himself and the world is different, and the quote from Bateson applies. Again, "It would appear that once precipitated into psychosis, the patient has a course to run. He is, as it were, embarked upon a voyage of discovery which is only completed by his return to the normal world to which he comes back with insights different from those of the inhabitants who never embarked on such a voyage. Once begun, a schizophrenic episode would appear to have as definite a course as an initiation ceremony-a death and rebirth-into which the novice may have been precipitated by his family life or by adventitious circumstances, but which in its course is largely steered by endogenous process".

Everyone that goes crazy, goes similarly. Each goes through similar kinds of experiences. The standard view that "psychosis" is bad is responsible for a lot of the treatment of the people said to be involved in this process. The misconception that if a person goes crazy, becomes schizophrenic, the disease is so bad that it justifies anything we do to stop the disease is a horribly punitive idea. We have punished the schizophrenic person over the ages by burning them at the stake; using dunking chairs; using various forms of electrical treatment; various forms of chemical poisons which vary from strychnine to Thorazine; locking them up for life; and psychosurgery—extricating vital parts of the brain.

Though some treatments of the past were harmful and cruel, many of the old treatments had only placebo effects. We do not use placebos today. Our drugs are carefully designed to alter psychological and physiological processes. The so-called side effects are, in fact, extensions of the wished for effects of the drugs. We use phenothiazines to block the actions of neurotransmitters in the limbic system to prevent thought transmissions. The drugs work in the sustantia nigra as well as in the rest of the limbic system and cause Parkinsonism. Thirty-five to fifty percent of the people given phenothiazines over a period of time will develop the incurable and serious condition called tardive dyskinesia. We give lithium to decrease the irritability of the nervous system by blocking the sodium-potassium shift necessary for nerve transmission. All the cells in the nervous system depend upon this mechanism for action. In the extreme, then, lithium functions as any other nerve poison, and causes death.

Being schizophrenic does not justify anything we care to do to the schizophrenic. If one looks into the process of people going through "enlightenment training" in Yoga, Zen, or even that of the Christian saints, one finds people being guided through this process. It seems that we need to be able to do the same, that is, guide those who find themselves in the process without having sought it.

Figure 7

Once a person has embarked upon this journey, going from normoid to normal, and has gotten into the world of "psychosis", (See Figure 7) and we get him back into his pre-morbid personality, there seems to be some pull back into the world of "psychosis". No matter what he or we do, the person is always going to get back into that world until he has completed the process of disorganization and reorganization. Perhaps he intuitively knows that normality is in having completed the process. Once the "I-Persona" no longer works, it will never work again. It is the Humpty-Dumpty story.

This, then, is the view of the "psychotic" process that I hold. When a person has had a breakdown, we are trying to see him through his breakdown, to support his disorganization and to facilitate his reorganization so that he does not have to go into the "psychotic" process over and over.

CHAPTER II: TREATMENT IMPLICATIONS OF VARIOUS ATTITUDES TOWARDS MENTAL ILLNESS

Mental illness is the term currently applied to a number of occurrences in the life of people. Historically, a variety of names have been applied to these occurrences. These include possession, madness, craziness, insanity, and nervous breakdown.

Mental illness has existed as part of the human condition since the beginning of recorded history, and we have every reason to believe that the very earliest man evidenced the same conditions that we call mental illness. Today, the term mental illness is generally understood, and the average person has some knowledge of the conditions encompassed by the term. For this reason, I will not attempt a rigorous definition. For my purposes, mental illness includes the neuroses, psychoses, and psychosomatic illness.

The main experiences of a person who undergoes a nervous breakdown are a change in the machinery of perception or a breakdown in the rational mind's ability to receive and combine perceptions and to make judgments from them. There is a sense of helplessness, together with a perfectly clear vision of one's helplessness and, most frequently, a degree of panic.

Mental illness appears in two main circumstances. The first is better known, but is the less frequently encountered. This is the breakdown that occurs when a person is overloaded by clearly apparent external stresses, such as combat fatigue and public or personal catastrophe. The second and more frequent circumstance is less well known. This is the breakdown that occurs when one has just reached some important goal in his life, such as graduation from school, purchase of one's dream house, or promotion to some long sought position. It is thought that in these latter circumstances, the person lets down his defenses and is overwhelmed by memories of the various struggles of his life.

The reactions of various societies to the person undergoing a mental illness have varied from time to time, and in some societies various reactions or attitudes towards mental illness have co-existed side by side.

The two main attitudes toward mental illness have been the religious or demonic and the scientific or medical. Both of these attitudes regard mental illness as bad and have led to the development of methods of exorcising or treating the condition. The degree of severity of the condition is used as a justification for whatever methods are used to bring it under control.

The demonic attitude states that the person who is mentally ill is sinful or in some way acting under the influence of demons which control him. In effect, the person's behavior is not his, but is the behavior of the demon or devil which possesses him. This attitude, which still exists in a lot of places, led to a variety of treatments.

Those treatments varied from incantations, tasks of various sorts, exhortations, prayers, exorcisms, and finally witch hunts and ultimately, in some cases, burnings. The idea was that witches were people whose possession was complete. It was estimated that tens of thousands of witches were killed before the practice of executing them ceased in 1782, when the last person was executed for witchcraft.

The second attitude, the scientific or medical one, is that the behaviors manifested by the person with mental illness are the result of chemical, viral, or other organic defects. Here again, the behavior is not the persons, but is the result of forces other than himself or his environment. This attitude has also led to a number of treatments. The mentally ill have been locked up and have been privileged to receive a number of different types of treatments in order to cure the illness.

These treatments have varied from exhortation to punishment. Some of them were in no way different from those used by the people who believed in evil spirits. For instance, dunking chairs and stocks were used by both religious and medical people. A variety of drugs were used, such as laxatives, sedatives, narcotics, strychnine, and other poisons. Starvation, bloodletting, cold showers, ice water baths, and hot packs have all been employed as treatment from time to time.

In the twentieth century, two modes of therapy, electroconvulsive or shock treatment and so-called psychosurgery, threatened to do for the medical attitude what burning witches did for the religious attitude. These two modes of treatment were worse that the illness. Both treatments caused permanent damage to the brain and, in many cases, wiped out the essence of the personality that made a person the distinct individual.

Faced with this dilemma, various psychiatrists began to revive an old attitude which regarded mental illness as a possible growth step in the life of man. As this attitude was enjoying some popularity in the late 1940s and early 1950s and promising to cause some real change in the methods of treating mental illness, a French drug company discovered a new class of chemicals which caused some changes in behavior. Specifically, these chemicals produced a bland, tranquil individual with, in the words of Henri Laborit, the discoverer, a "disinterest in all that goes on around him".

These drugs did control the signs of mental illness and were not thought to cause permanent damage. The loss of spontaneity, creativity, and the emotional spark of life was considered a small price to pay to stamp out mental illness. However, contrary facts were soon to be discovered. These drugs, the highly heralded phenothiazines, are selective biological poisons and have detrimental effects on the human brain, which are permanent and apparently irreversible.

In the late 1960s, another biological poison, lithium carbonate, was introduced into medicine. A substance found in the waters in European spas, it had fallen into disrepute because of the deaths of several people who had "taken too much of the waters." It does cause a person to be tranquil, however, and with very careful control, extremely serious effects can be avoided, we think. However, it is unreasonable to believe that a drug which poisons all the sodium containing chemical systems in the body can fail to cause very serious long-term problems.

It really seems that people who hold the attitude that mental illness is a disease have advanced only to the point reached by the advocates of the evil-spirit attitude. Namely, the cure is worse than the disease.

An answer to this dilemma possibly lies in the third attitude towards mental illness, namely that the set of changes we call mental illness are in fact a growth sign and can lead a person to a more mature state of awareness and more competent functioning.

A person may develop a set of coping skills to deal with life situations and learn to use these skills so very well that they are relied upon to the exclusion of other skills which are not fully developed. When, for some reason, the situation changes, the only skills which are fully developed are those which do not apply to the new situation. But the person continues to respond with these developed skills, and anxiety and feelings of helplessness increase until the person begins to search for new skills or methods. If this process is allowed to continue and not interfered with by extreme measures, it can be a growth process resulting in a person who is more integrated, has a more extensive selection of coping skills, and is more capable of dealing with his changing life situation.

An analogy might be found in the redecorating of a room. A degree of disorder and disarray is necessary as old furnishings and decorations are removed or rearranged and new furnishings and decorations are brought in.

There is a large body of literature from a number of cultures to support this point of view. In child development, it is known that there is a period of turmoil in the child as he progresses from one stage to another. This turmoil can at time look like mental illness. It is, in fact, the disorganization of old and outgrown modes of coping prior to organization of more adaptive methods. Gail Sheehy in *Passages* details the crisis of adult life and describes a number of cases in which people went through full-blown psychotic episodes in moving from one stage of development into middle age. She indicates that if a person is not allowed to complete the process of transition in other developmental stages, changes during the middle age crisis will be more abrupt and disorganizing than if the person had been allowed to progress through each of the previous stage changes smoothly.

A number of psychiatrists have again begun to consider the validity of this point of view. The psychiatrist's interest in the turmoil that accompanies conflict resolution was evident before the advent of the phenothiazine tranquilizers. Now, with the realization that these drugs, as well as their successors the so-called atypicals are so dangerous, psychiatrists are again considering the possibility that we need to learn other methods of helping people through these changes rather than drugging them or subjecting them to other destructive methods of treatment.

Some methods which have been used as alternative treatments are intensive psychotherapy in a protective environment, such as a psychiatric ward, relaxation techniques, family therapy, meditation, exercise and massage. These treatments are designed to help the mentally ill person to regain control of his mental faculties and to see his condition as a growth experience which can help him to better relate to himself his family, and his community as well as help him to better live in the complex world with which we all have to cope.

CHAPTER III: DEPRESSION

This has been called the age of depression. The diagnosis of depression is made quite often, and the most frequently prescribed medicines are for depression. There are two types of depression. Hermann Hesse describes depression as follows in his novel, *Steppenwolf*:

"The day had gone by just as days go by. I had killed it in accordance with my primitive and retiring way of life. I had worked for an hour or so in perusing pages of old books. I had had pains for two hours, as elderly people do. I had taken a powder and had been very glad when the pains consented to disappear. I had lain in a hot bath and had absorbed its kindly warmth. Three times the mail had come with undesired letters and circulars to look through. I had done my breathing exercises. I had been for an hour's walk and seen the loveliest feathery cloud pattern penciled against the sky. That was very delightful, so was the reading of the old books, so was lying in the warm bath. But taken all in all, it had not been exactly a day of rapture. No, it had not even been a day brightened with happiness and joy. Rather, it had been just one of those days which for a long while now had fallen to my lot. The moderately pleasant and holy, bearable and tolerable lukewarm days of a discontented middle-aged man. Days without special pain, without special cares, without particular worry, without despair, days when I calmly wonder, objective and fearless, whether it isn't time to follow the example of a Delbert Stiekler and have an accident while shaving. He who has known the other days, the angry ones of gout attacks or those with that wicked headache rooted behind the eyeballs that cast a spell on every nerve of eye and ear with a fiendish delight; and torture or soul destroying evil days of inward vacancy and despair. When on this distracted earth, sucked dry by the vampires of finance, the world of man and of so-called culture grins back at us with a lying, vulgar, brazen, glamour of affair, and dogs us with a persistence of an emetic. When all is concentrated and focused to the last pitch of the intolerable, upon our

"

own sick self, he who has known these days of hell may be content indeed with normal half and half days like today."

That quote is a very artistic description by a person suffering from neurotic depression, and having insight into his condition, as contrasted to the person with psychotic depression. The depressive process is one that finds its roots early in childhood for most people who suffer from it, but which may find its beginnings later in life. What follows is my view of the depressive process. My approach is that of a clinician as opposed to that of a researcher. A joke tells the difference between the two: "A clinician and a researcher are included in a study by another researcher. The researcher conducting the study wants these two men to complete a task. He puts them at one end of a hall, and at the other end of the hall, he puts a beautiful nude woman. He says to his subjects, 'I want you to go to her and I want you to go by dividing the distance in half each time.' The researcher says, 'We will never be able to get there.' The clinician says, 'Yeah, but we will be able to get close enough.'" The approach I present is close enough for now.

The passage from *Steppenwolf,* by Hermann Hesse describes two types of depression. The vague kind of dysphoria that goes with one kind, and the hard, physical, almost concrete type of depression that goes with the other type. The following framework for understanding the two types of depression is drawn in part from *The Attitudinal Theory of Emotion*, by Nina Bull. Ms. Bull worked at Columbia University. I also draw on the work of Dr. James Papez, who formulated the concept of the Papez circuits based on his work on the limbic system in the brain. Dr. Paul D. McLean, who worked at NIMH, has elaborated further the work on the limbic system. I include these ideas to attempt to move to a more concrete idea of depression, and away from some of the abstract formulations.

The Attitudinal Theory of Emotion proposes that emotion is based on bodily sets or attitudes. It has been known since the time of Aristotle that there is a preparatory phase for all action. If one is going to strike, he has to form a platform from which to launch his strike. That forming of the platform is the assumption of an attitude or a posture or of a position which indicates action. If an incoming stimulus provokes an attitude and action follows directly, there is no emotion. If the time line between the attitude and the action is long, there is emotion. As humans, we have the capacity to delay action, and most frequently do. Then we have feelings, which are cortical interpretations of the proprioceptive and enteroceptive inputs into the hypothalamus, and subsequently the cortex.

A stimulus occurs, and attitude is assumed, and then there is a delay. During the time delay, the organism is ready. He is prepared to do something. We then feel the state of our organism, to feel how we are. We can measure the state of our organism by external means, such as EKG, EMG, and GSR.

There are four negative emotions. Many words are used to describe emotions, but they can be factored into these four. For instance, one can say that he is irritated, a little irritated, a lot irritated, but irritation factors into the emotion anger. The four negative emotions are sadness, anger, disgust, and fear. Sadness is the feeling that one gets when he has assumed an attitude of crying and has not cried, but has inhibited that expression. Anger is a readiness to attack, inhibited. Disgust is the emotion that we have when we assume the attitude of vomiting and inhibit that action. Fear is the emotion we get when we inhibit the action of fleeing.

Disgust is one of the most important and deep of the feelings. It is also called dislike by Ms. Bull and by the Silvan S. Tomkins and the affective theorists. Many taboos are based on this emotion. To inhibit vomiting, we turn our heads and hold our breath. This inhibits the motility of the gut through connections to the sympathetic nervous system.

There are two types of behavior: goal-directed and obstacle-directed. Goal directed behavior is that behavior that occurs as we follow our inclinations towards a goal. We are forwards looking, focused, moving. Our organisms are balanced, and we have no interference, for instance, with our binocular vision. The work we have to do to achieve the goal is perceived as part of the goal. Goal directed behavior generates a healthy sense of making progress and of having an aim. One feels "together" or integrated.

Goals are usually set based on our biological needs. If we feel hunger, we set food as a goal. A hypothetically healthy person sets his goals based upon his perception of his internal state and his previous experiences and on the availability of that which might satisfy his needs. The hungry person who desires a steak might be satisfied with a hamburger if steaks are too hard to come by.

Obstacle-directed behavior occurs if a person is proceeding towards a goal and encounters something that blocks his forward progress. The obstacle is something that is not overcome by the person's repertoire of behaviors. It stands between him and the goal. It looms larger than the goal. It blocks his forward progress despite his attempts to overcome it. It represents an extraordinary event. If one wants to build a piece of furniture, getting of wood is not considered an obstacle. If the work is considered an obstacle, the person is showing obstacle-directed behavior and is depressed. Young people often tell me of a goal, such as becoming a physician, and quickly follow that statement with one indicating that the length of study, etc., get in their way. That is an example of an obstacle orientation, often of a chronic nature.

An obstacle in a person free from the chronic obstacle orientation generates emotion, thought, and problem solving. Once the person has gotten the obstacle out of the way, or has grieved for the goal, he is free of emotion, and free to continue towards his goal or to set other goals. If problem solving behavior does not work, the person might lapse into frustration and depression. Several episodes of such failure might result in the person internalizing the obstacle orientation and lapsing into habitual obstacle-oriented behavior any time he meets with a difficult or new situation.

The obstacles that affect us most strongly are the attempts to be pleasing to the significant persons in our lives, most frequently those people upon whom we have projected our dependency or nurturance needs. If such a person becomes an obstacle for us, our own needs become reasons for not dealing with the obstacle. We often invoke the defense mechanisms of denial, repression, etc., to prevent ourselves from knowing what is happening in our lives.

In such cases, there is the development of a frustrational complex. Here the obstacle is large, the goal is not surrenderable, either because of its intrinsic value of the symbolic value attached to it. At this point, the person feels a lot of emotional turmoil. The state of being frustrated becomes fixated. The person has the capacity to abstract and to identify his feelings. Since emotions are complex, the person usually feels more than one of them. He then moves to giving up. The person may then move to a point of incapacity, passivity, a blunting of emotional behavior, and then he is depressed. Depression contains a mixture of grievance, protest, complaint over the primary frustration and constitutes an even more perplexing obstacle to the organism because it is internal. The obstacle, whatever it was, is lost sight of. He is at this point fixated upon his own attitudes and internal states. If the obstacle is someone he first knew that he was angry at, or disgusted at, or afraid of, or he was very sad because that person would not get out of his way or perform a task for him, or whatever, then there was an orientation towards that person, or an identification with that person. This latter may be identification with the aggressor. The obstacle may be a drunken parent, and one can become so fixated as to drink to excess. In the progression into depression, the fixation is on the attitudes within the person. These vague feelings sometimes progress to rigid feelings of helplessness in the person and become totally immobile in a psychotically depressed patient.

When the person is a depressed mother, the children around her may organize to try to get her to moving. If this does not work, and the child is left without a functional mother, he may become quite depressed himself.

Depression and the various preceding states are visible in the attitudes of the person. Emotional states leave their sets in the body of the person. At the deepest level, these neuromuscular states called attitudes must be changed for the person to achieve freedom from them. (See my paper *Mind-Body Integration.*)

Goals are set by the brain stem. There are three divisions which mediate the behavior of the person. Those have to do with self-survival, species survival, and the survival of the social group. The first division involves drives for nurturance, food, water, and air. The second has to do with sex and a place to do it (territory), and the third has to do with hierarchy, status, and social standing. Behaviors mediated by the first division are a search for the nurturing other, the separation cry, food seeking, eating, drinking, breathing, etc. The behaviors mediated by the second division involve courtship, mating, establishing territory, etc. The behaviors mediated by the third division are dominance-submission, group recognition, display, etc. and are connected with the symbol-driven part of the cortex.

Depression in children result from unmet needs from the first division, from unmet dependency needs. The motivating force of the child is self-preservation. He strives to find fit with the nurturing or caretaking other so that he will be fed, cleaned, warmed, and protected. When he is frustrated in this, he may go through a series of behaviors before lapsing into despair and depression. Jane Goodall described a situation from her experience in studying primates in which the mother of a baby monkey died suddenly. The baby monkey tried to get her mother to moving. She tried over and over before giving up, assuming a dejected and morose posture. The little monkey finally died itself. This type of behavior occurs in modified form in the children of depressed mothers.

To treat depression, one must help the person to examine his life, as in the case of the children above. He can then see his needs, identify the obstacles, and begin to work towards achieving his needs or do necessary grieving.

The therapist must recognize that feelings are based on an external reality and strive to help the patients to get beyond the "ego defenses" and evaluate his reality. Denial is not a river.

CHAPTER IV: BIOLOGY OF RELATIONAL SYSTEMS

A general social-systems premise is that psychiatric symptoms may not only be a reaction to the environment, but also an implicit, nonverbal, and veiled criticism of the environment. This is in contrast to the prevailing biological reductionistic theory that psychiatric symptoms originate in genetically determined disorders of transmitters within the single synapse. In the latter theory, there can be no heuristic value in psychiatric symptoms and professionals holding to that theory blame the patient's body rather than looking for the cause of the symptoms in human predicaments. Though the biological reductionistic theory holds the center stage, its proponents are losing the battle to help those who find themselves unable to function in modern society. At the same time, the social-systems theorists have not been able to integrate the findings of biology into their theories, and often seem abstract in their descriptions.

This paper is an attempt to move towards a more concrete system of understanding of the symptoms seen in a number of psychiatric disorders. These disorders include autism, obsessive compulsive disorder, anxiety disorders, and the psychoses. I will include a brief discussion of the emergence of a new clinical picture variously called "the young chronic," "MICA" or mentally ill chemically addicted, dual diagnosis patients, or "social breakdown syndrome." This syndrome might better be called "anomic turmoil" based on the concept of "anomie" introduced by Durkheim in 1897. Durkheim held that when a society is in a state of disarray with an absence of norms or laws by which to guide behavior or when an individual can find no niche within the status quo, suicide becomes a more likely occurrence. This approach to the etiology of suicide emphasizes that lack of integration into a functional social order is devastating to mental health.

The relational system is central to the presence of a functional social order. The relational system includes structures within the central nervous system which are included in the genes of the species and is observable in the attachment behavior of the newborn and his mother. Though Freud understood that schizophrenia was caused by a pre-oedipal disturbance, and later analysts understood the impact of the intrusive, unempathic mother who violated the child's ego-boundaries, it was the direct observations of Bowlby and Ainsworth who gave us our understanding of the effect of failures in the bonding process between the mother and the child.

Bowlby observed the attachment patterns of toddlers, finding two types of deviation from normal bonding. Those were the alienated behavior of those youngsters who paid little heed to their mother's comings-and-goings, as compared to the clinging attachments of those youngsters who could hardly let their mothers out of their sight. Bowlby perceived the former group in terms of "maternal deprivation." Those children seemed unable to maintain stable bonds to anyone and ultimately were prone to antisocial behavior. In contrast, the latter group were seen as having difficulties with separation-individuation. Those children had been subjected to "smother love" and were considered susceptible to neurosis and in extreme cases to schizophrenia.

Ainsworth, a student of Bowlby, studied children at age one and again identified two major deviations from the usual innate propensity toward attachment. The first was an under-attached, aggressive, and noncompliant "avoidant" group. The second was an over-attached, easily frustrated, and less competent "anxious/ambivalent" group. Ainsworth then traced the impact of each early deviation on adult adjustment and found extension beyond childhood to subsequent dealing with relatives, friends, and mates. She noted that the attachment pattern organized during the first year of life becomes an internal model for relationships that serves as a template for subsequent adult relationships. Be reminded of this as we discuss the "no-parent family."

These observations have been supported by various family therapists, though there has not yet emerged a coherent set of theories which include the multiple levels of observations that have been done. At the current time, the field of family therapy has modified its systems approach to state that the individual "disappears" within a composite family ego-mass, but the behavior of each member continues to be viewed within a context of family interdependence and enmeshment.

The work of Paul D. MacLean helps us to further understand the relationship system. MacLean's work is summarized in his book, *The Triune Brain in Evolution*, published in 1989. The following is an attempt at a clinical application of this important research.

MacLean's work moves beyond the observation of dyads to a phylogenetic perspective. He noted that within each human being are three brains: the reptilian, the paleomammalian and the neomammalian. The reptilian brain as it exists in lizards is such that the lizard is hatched with all the abilities for survival except procreation. The goals set by humans are set in the reptilian brain. These include three classes of behavior: (1) nurturance or feeding and other self-preservation skills; (2) sex and a place to do it, i.e., territoriality; and (3) social activities such as formation of social groups, flocking, migration or preservation of the social order.

The paleomammalian brain or limbic system is a "border around" the brain stem structures and modulates the basic drives so that the early mammals could engage in nursing in conjunction with maternal care, audio vocal communication for maintaining maternal-offspring contact and play to serve harmony in the nest.

With the incorporation of a large part of the neomammalian brain into the limbic system, the third division has come to be involved with activities such as status and hierarchy and the symbols for them and the feelings generated by such symbols. The limbic system structures are in the main designed to modulate behavior so that sucking and the prolonged extra corporeal maturation of the mammals can occur. Lizards eat their young, so modulation of feeding patterns is necessary for mothers to suckle their young. The mother must not eat her young and the infant must also quickly learn to modulate his feeding urges to fit into the social structure of his species. At the same time, some form of recognition of one's specific offspring is necessary. In reindeer herds, for instance, a calf who wanders too far from its mother will die, despite the presence of a number of lactating females. The mother can recognize her own calf's cry from among a large number of calves in the herd.

In the neomammalian brain, the increase in the cingulate gyrus and the incorporation of the prefrontal cortex and the change towards vision as the dominant guiding sense has enabled a very varied number of patterns for child rearing. This has no parallel in the reptilian brain. The progression towards visual and symbolic expression reaches its highest point in man. This is the area that is trained as we learn the symbolic and verbal cues which allow us to function in a complex society. Hamsters without a neocortex grow normally, go through daily routines, mate, breed and successfully rear their young and develop play behavior at the appropriate age. Extirpation of the cingulate gyrus causes deficits in maternal behavior, including deficits in nest building, nursing and pup retrieval.

A summary of the brain function is as follows: goals are set by the brain stem. The three classes of goals are: (1) feeding and nurturance seeking and fighting for self-preservation (rage); (2) sex and territoriality with its goal-directed fighting; and, finally, (3) status and belonging. These three classes of goals are organized and modulated in a species specific way by the three divisions of the limbic system. The primary mode of function of the limbic system is inhibition of the drives initiated in the brain stem and integration of the emotions which follow as a result of this inhibition. The third division is associated with language and is trained in the child-rearing process. Its primary purpose was to maintain the mother-child contact and to modulate behavior to allow for suckling and to mediate sounds for mother-child contact and eventually to modulate play to preserve harmony in the nest. Later symbolic functions included clan preservation, status and organization of hunting and defense parties, etc. The third division of the limbic system allows for cooperative endeavors between members of hunting groups by its control of the more primal hierarchy producing drives of the lower primates, for instance, and for community living; however, a lot of training must occur. Training demands the presence of another person.

Bonding or the feeling of belonging necessitates a constant other, as shown by Bowlby. Further along, separation-individuation must occur. The consistent other must be there, but must also have a sense of self: me-not me, and teach the child the gestalt "no-no", which is the symbolic boundary setter. Without a sense of me-not me, the child will be unable to function with others.

In the extreme, this failure to teach the "no-no" gestalt results in the child who is totally unable to explore his environment: the autistic child who cannot use speech, who is so afraid of his environment that he does repetitive motions, and who goes into a rage when he is attracted to an object in his environment. This child is so tentative in his relationships with others that he often seems to be treating them as things. He often clings to his mother's body much as a baby monkey clings to his mother. At the same time, the mothers of these children seem to have no clear idea about where the mother ends and the child starts and the difference between the mother's needs and the needs of the child. Interestingly, the mother often gets her dependency and nurturance needs met through the people upon whom she makes demands for the care of her child.

Further along the spectrum is the obsessive compulsive person, whose uncertainty leads him to extreme inhibition of action, with an attendant intensification of emotion which cannot be discharged in fantasy nor play. The descriptions in *"So the Witch Won't Eat Me" Fantasy and the Child's Fear of Infanticide,* by Dorothy Bloch, are helpful in understanding the effect of witnessing violence or by occasionally being its target in an environment where the hope of being loved had not been completely extinguished.

The hyperactive or limit-seeking child is another victim of the poor training which can result from deficiencies in the relational system. Since this child does not know where he stops nor starts and does not have the "no-no" gestalt, he is continually looking for the limits in the situation. He does not know that a rule to sit in the chair is limiting of his permission to get up. He does not know that the rule to read from left-to-right limits the movement of his eyes. Since his mother was not seen as a limit setter, nor a rule maker, no other authority figure is seen as such. This drives teachers, the quintessential rule makers, crazy as it does other authority figures.

In the early characterization of schizophrenia, there was thought to be a failure of separation-individuation due to family enmeshment. The new schizophrenic or "young chronic," though, is a person who is characterized by fragmented bonds and inconsolable object-seeking due to disruptions in attachments. The family has changed from a nuclear family with a mother overly involved with her children to the "one-parent" family to the "no-parent" family. Though the mother may be present, Rutter has observed that poor quality of care rather than absence or death constitute the most disturbing neglect for the child. In this context, the new schizophrenia has emerged, characterized by character disorder, cognitive slippage and substance abuse. This patient's non-compliance, aggression and addiction, along with demands for immediate attention and instant relief make them unpopular with treatment personnel.

Ainsworth was careful to state that the traits arising from disturbances in the attachment system during the first year of life were not fixed in infancy, but could be modified by altered maternal behavior or relevant life events. Herein lies the problem with the reductionistic method. Our attempt has been to devise a "feel-good" pill so good that patients (and non-patients) can function in even the most noxious and abusive situations without any distress. This ignores the systems precept that for meaningful change to occur, it must be at a level above the expression of the symptom. Some examples of change at a level above the symptom follow.

In the case of the autistic child, we must work with the mother to help her to appreciate the difference between her needs and her body and the needs and the body of the child. We must help her to see the child's exploratory behavior as normal and to allow it after she has taught him that her body is a "no-no." With the obsessive-compulsive child or adult, we must get him to act on his desires, rather than suppressing them. This necessitates alteration of parental attitudes and practices in treating children and confrontation of the internalized parental attitudes in treating the adult. With the hyperactive child, we must work with the family to help them to teach the child the meaning of the "no-no" gestalt, rather than continually punishing him or conversely excusing him on the basis of some putative defect in his body. With the new chronic, we must practice early detection and institute the proper treatment within the relational system. This latter might recognize that changes in the larger society rather than within the family are necessary.

Specifically to the family therapists, I recommend that we integrate into our theories the existing knowledge of the biology of the relational system. Then we must confront the reductionistic approach which has become the cry of the psychiatric profession, the third-party payers, and often of families who had rather the pathology be in the body of the patient rather than in the way the family lives and in the society which has little use for self-criticism.

CHAPTER VI: AIKIDO AND MIND-BODY INTEGRATION

In 1967, after four years in the General Practice of Medicine, I started a residency in Psychiatry. A large percentage of my general practice patients suffered from psychiatric conditions and I read psychiatric literature voraciously, as I did during my first year of residency. I became more and more mystified during that year, as we were presented with so many systems of psychology and psychiatry, each of which, taken by itself, seemed to "make sense." Taken together, those systems seemed conflicting and confusing. During a discussion of this confusion with my brother, then a graduate student in speech and communications, he suggested I learn about an epistemology called General Semantics. After I followed his suggestion, and applied Korzybski's principles about abstracting to my studies, my confusion cleared remarkably. I enjoyed teaching those principles to students, residents, preceptees, patients, etc., over the years. It was always fun to see the comprehension bloom when I could get a student to sit long enough with a person overwhelmed, for instance, by a quandary without diagnosing or classifying so he could see the person and help him clarify his situation and arrive at a workable solution.

I discovered my second passion in 1974. That summer, my family and I spent our vacation in an isolated lake cabin. I ate a lot, fished, and read potboilers. One of those books featured a hero who used Aikido to deal with bad guys. I had a book on Aikido in my library and got it out as soon as I returned home. Serendipitously, in September of that year, Dr. Greg Faulkner moved to my hometown of Huntsville, Alabama, to work in the space industry. He started an Aikido Class, which I joined. I have practiced since then and taught for a number of those years.

My general sense of well-being began to improve soon after starting Aikido. My body habitus changed and people remarked that I moved more freely. When one of my psychiatric colleagues attended a trial workshop, I remarked to him that Aikido had intrinsic value different from other martial arts, and different from the attendant exercise. He did not agree, and I was unable to defend my point. A number of years later, the acknowledged best fighter in our federation of martial artists, an engineer, wondered why we all continued to practice martial arts over the years. I have attempted to answer the question about the intrinsic value of Aikido, as I believe there is such, and also the question of why I continue to practice and to teach the art. I think it is a tool to help me "make sense", especially in the face of confrontational, aggressive persons.

The human ability to conceptualize and objectify accounts for many of our accomplishments. This ability also accounts for one of the major problems that we have to solve: a dichotomy between one's subjective or organic self and an "I-Persona" or "I-Mask" self-concept. We describe ourselves on currency subject to being overvalued and vulnerable to being blown away by the wind of events, leaving us with a diminished sense of self-worth. In this paper, I will explore this split and in particular how the practice of the Japanese martial art of Aikido helps to resolve this problem.

This split occurs as part of development. In normal development there is a reorganization of the conceptual framework to fit the reality of the person and his world at the end of each stage of development. There is a period of turmoil associated with this state of reorganization that must be tolerated and supported by the environment. Since most human environments do not support any kind of turmoil, few people have been able to complete this part of each stage of development. For that reason, most people have a mixture of out-of-date ideas and conclusions in their conceptual frameworks.

Charles Kelly wrote that there are two character types based on two different ways of conceptualizing: the mechanic and the mystic. The first, the mechanic, operates in concepts, deals with the world by means of discrete units, and treats the world as though it is fundamentally static and immobile. He acts and operates on an outside reality to the exclusion of subjectivity or consciousness. The mystic over-focuses on the subjective "feeling" aspect of the life process at the expense of the objective "action" aspect. He becomes convinced that subjective reality antedates and overrides the merely physical reality of the body and the external world. He develops the conviction that consciousness is independent of the body.

In his essay on metaphysics, Bergson wrote, "There is an absolute knowledge, which can only be given in an intuition (meaning coming only from an internal processing). Everything else falls within the province of analysis," i.e., the world of the mechanic and the mystic. "By intuition is meant the kind of intellectual sympathy by which one places oneself within an object in order to coincide with what is unique in it and consequently inexpressible. There is a reality that is external and yet given immediately to the mind." I think this is inherent in the "staying at the level of nonverbal" talked about in General Semantics.

Alfred Korzybski, who originated General Semantics, called this level of the intuitive the level of the nonverbal: the level of being and knowing without the use of symbols or words. He recommended that one stay at the level of the nonverbal until he comes to a complete knowledge and acceptance of a situation. We have to use words and symbols to communicate; however, being able to stay at the level of the nonverbal until we have contacted the external reality is important. This ability increases the reliability of our abstracting process by allowing us to gather more information before arriving at conclusions, inferences, etc.

These concepts relate to my work as a psychiatrist in that practically every person has a concept of self quite different from what can be seen or perceived in that person. People define themselves according to their status, their role, what they have been told about themselves years ago or out-of-date self-definitions. These same people often have a conceptualization of external reality that is eccentric and cannot be consensually validated. Psychotherapy, when done right, helps the person get to a sense of reality of self and helps him develop a consensually validatable conceptualization of external reality.

Aikido is another way a person can develop a more accurate perception of self and a more nearly accurate conceptualization of external reality. In Aikido there is a particular necessity of evaluating reality accurately.

Aikido is a modern martial art originated in Japan by Morihei Uyeshiba, called by Aikidoists O-Sensei or The Great Teacher (of Aikido of course). Morihei Uyeshiba was a seeker who started out early in life with a decision that he would never get beaten up. He had seen his father bullied by village ruffians and made the decision that he would not be such a victim. He entered into the study of martial arts as a young man, studying the way of the sword and the way of the empty hand, Jujitsu, and eventually ending up in a martial art called Daito Jujitsu. He was an undefeated fighter. He was capable with a sword or an empty hand of beating practically anybody in a fight and took great pride in his ability. He was sergeant-at-arms for a spiritual sect, and later a hand-to-hand combat instructor for the Japanese Navy. With all of those skills under his command, he came into conflict with a close friend, a naval officer who was a professor of fencing.

Consider the paradox. Uyeshiba was a man who said he would never be beaten up and who had taken great pride in fighting and his ability to fight. He now confronted a friend who had attacked him with a wooden sword to kill him. He was faced with a situation in which his self-identification conflicted with an external and intuitively felt reality. When does your friend become your enemy? How can you kill your friend? Morihei Uyeshiba fought this "battle" with the naval officer by using only defensive moves. When the naval officer moved to strike, Uyeshiba would move out of the way. He continued to do evasive tactics until the opponent collapsed in a sweat. Then Uyeshiba went out into the garden where he experienced a sense of lights and a revelation about the martial arts. This revelation was that martial arts are not to kill and destroy your enemy but to restore harmony that has been previously disturbed in the universe. From this experience, he formulated a new conceptualization of *Budo* or the Way of War.

Uyeshiba's conceptualization was based in part on the actual meaning of the Japanese character "Bu". The idea is that an individual stops war or fighting. The top of the character is of two crossed halberds, indicating a cessation of aggressiveness. The lower character literally means to stop. The composite, therefore, would imply "to stop fighting" or end battle. He originally called his method of self-defense Aiki-jujitsu and later renamed it Aikido. *Aiki* means harmony of the energies. The word *do*, which means Way in the spiritual sense, added to aiki forms Aikido that means the way of harmony of the energies. Aikido is the current designation of the Way of Morihei Uyeshiba.

In addition to being an extremely effective form of self-defense, Aikido became a basis for the pursuit of the true self. This pursuit is done by the constant reevaluation (mind) in the learning and application of the techniques of Aikido (body). In order to do Aikido effectively, one has to cultivate an awareness of the body, the location of the body in space and the force of his movements. This constant reevaluation ideally caused a shift from the concept of opponents, as in self-defense, to partners, who would help in rediscovering the true self. Consequently he was "making sense" of a previously perceived paradox. His martial skills remained the same, or improved, but the application changed from aggressiveness to cooperation (or in the words of Trigant Burrow from ditention to contention).

The philosophy of Aikido is the culmination of a philosophy that had required centuries of evolution and was very much a part of the life of the samurai. The first step in this evolution was that of the samurai or servant warrior. He belonged to his master and if ordered, his job was to kill the enemy. The samurai learned that this kind of killing is spiritual suicide. Then came the concept of mutual destruction, i.e., of sacrificing one's life to kill the enemy. In that situation, a sense of appreciation of one's life emerged. It is no sacrifice if your life is valueless. Then evolved the concept of the mutual preservation of life, the idea of the saving of one's enemy's life while preserving one's own life. The warrior must have a profound knowledge of his craft in order to actualize a philosophy of saving his and his enemy's life. Otherwise he has no choice other than to kill or be killed. His knowledge must not be of a mechanical nor of a mystical nature, i.e., abstractions have no place when one is faced with an enemy skilled in the art of killing and determined to end his life. The warrior's knowledge must be based on an intuitive perception of movement and forces. It was out of the background of the Zen considerations of the samurai that Morihei Uyeshiba was able to have his enlightenment experience from which he developed his Aikido, "The Way of Harmony."

In the world we certainly have to be able to deal with aggression that arises in many contexts. When we are afraid we will often retire into the world of thoughts and fantasies. The Aikidoist must learn the skills of containing his emotions in situations where the threat is only symbolic. When the attack is physical, however, and only then, the Aikidoist has a place to "enter the spirit" of the attacker and neutralize the attack. The skills that are necessary for self-defense can be demonstrated, but must be learned through constant practice. The first of these skills is to avoid opposition. This means blending with the attack, redirecting it, etc. The second is to neutralize further aggression with techniques such as locks and throws.

Aikido practice is a different experience for most students from about any other activity. In a safe, non-competitive environment, he is able to practice dealing with physical aggression. The usual verbal world does not apply so strongly. If the student is hit, he is hurt. That knowledge does not come to the student mathematically. He does not go to his computer to calculate the trajectory, velocity, or the mass of a fist. By the time he even thinks those thoughts, he will have felt his practice partner's controlled punch. Intuitively the student learns that if he is not there when a blow arrives, he is, for an instant, okay. He is not okay forever because his attacker may have a variety of other attacks available, but the student is okay for the very present instant of time that is the only one he has. In this process the student learns to appreciate the here and now, the present moment. He must then develop skills that make his attacker fail in subsequent attacks, and must be able to sequence his defensive techniques in order to have a coherent personal self-defense. The student thereby develops an intuitive knowledge of time.

In this process, something happens to the student. He gets out of the abstract, out of the world of conceptualization, whether it is mechanical or mystical. Though the student may be trained in biophysics and be able to do intricate calculations, as long as he is doing those calculations he is not in the world as it exists at that moment. The student may be a mystical adept, but no amount of consciousness separate from action can keep him from being struck. The student practicing Aikido correctly has moved out of his mind and into his self, into his perceptions and intuition, and has developed an effective way of action.

An example of this transition can be found in a student who came to my class. One of my favorite students kept mentioning his best friend, who wanted to come to class, but was afraid, and was "a little strange." He finally came. He would have fit into the category of persons formerly called "simple schizophrenic" with his reticence, lack of touch with his body, etc. I learned that he, at age 25, had three two-year certificates from our local junior college. He had read widely, and I was to learn, could discuss the books he read. He had never had a job, did not have a driver's license. He had had some very dangerous experiences hitch-hiking around the country alone. In class, he had little positional sense, had difficulty with tasks requiring agility, and requiring perception of the actions of a training partner. He persisted, though, and slowly learned to do Aikido rolls, punch, avoid a punch, and learned his beginner techniques. He went to a weeklong workshop with the class. At the end of that week, he had made friends with students from other classes.

When our group met to decide if we would stay for the closing party, he was very quiet. When I insisted on his input, he verbalized that he had made friends, and wanted to party with them. The others of us who had attended a number of such parties acquiesced. His eyes filled with tears, and he said that he had never been asked for his preference before. As time went on, he got a girlfriend, a job, bought a car that his girlfriend used to take him to his job, which, by the way conflicted with Aikido practice. He was studying for his driver's license when I last saw him.

Another example can be found in a young woman, the epitome of the "Southern Belle" who came to class to be with her boyfriend, an accomplished Aikidoist. We were practicing an especially hard throw that required her to be different from her usual demure self. She would do a couple of throws or be thrown hard, break into tears, sit out for a moment or two and then reenter practice. It was great over time to see her become less tentative and less appeasing. She quit, as we used to say, trying to "sweet her way through life".

Motion is a metaphysical idea. It is not something one can deal with on his computer, especially if there is a fist coming toward his nose. The student must act and not be where the fist is going. A transformation in his way of being must occur. He can then walk around amongst men and not be totally afraid because his skills are such that he does not have to pull his .38, blow someone's brains out and go to jail or impoverish himself spiritually. He can deal with aggression in a controlled and rational way, without having to go to the ultimate.

There is another thing that happens. There are reflexes in the human body that are elicited, for instance, when a person is choked. At the instant of this severe assault, the reflexive action is to freeze. Human beings are neither fighters nor runners; we are freezers. If a person has gone beyond the reflex, he is able to apply carefully developed techniques of self-defense. He can then render the attacker powerless.

In gathering Aikido skills, we correct the split between the Conceptual Self and the True Self. The movement into the body gives one an opportunity to find and correct attitudes and integrate stored body memories. When a person is moving and has gone back into the intuition about self, he can feel things in himself, in his body where experiences are stored.

A personal example of this is found in an experience of mine on the mat. We were practicing defenses against chokes in an especially intense workout. I found myself frozen, unable to practice, and somewhat emotional. I followed our practice of sitting out on the side of the mat. I had a visual memory of an event that occurred in my early teens. An uncle visiting in my home and I were bantering. The jibes became somewhat cruel, and I responded by mentioning a sore point of my uncle's. He went into a rage and attacked me by grabbing me around the neck with his hands. My chair went over, and he was on top of me choking me. I may have been killed, had not my father intervened. I remembered the event without the emotions until that point on the Aikido mat, and thought the event had been solved, but was always leery of anyone I thought to be potentially explosive. Following that, my comfort with others improved considerably.

This, then, is the Way, the Aikido, the leading away from the conceptual and back to the real. At the same time that one is developing an extremely effective self-defense, he is confronting some of the inhibitions and prohibitions that he has stored in his body under the direction of the limbic system, and finding ways of bringing them into awareness so that they can be integrated into the functioning Self.

If one has at his command such an effective defense against aggression, he is able to stay at the nonverbal longer even in the face of a bellicose bullying other, and allow his thinking to move towards a solution. In Aikido, one moves toward the True Self subjectively perceived, intuitively felt. One integrates the reality as examined by the senses and derives concepts from this process so that goals are set from the perception of one's internal states and then sought freely without the prohibitions and inhibitions that we tend to build into ourselves.

Curtis L.V. Adams, M.D., Shichidan
Midori Yama Budokai Aikido

APPENDIX: MEDITATION

(Psychophysiological Integration)

1. Sit comfortably.

2. Fix your eyes on a point across the room.

3. Become aware of sensations around your eyes.

4. Your breathing changes.

5. Become aware of tensions in parts of your body other than around your eyes.

6. Your thinking changes.

7. Your tensions go away.

Twenty minutes morning and night is recommended. A timer is helpful. A straight-backed chair with arms is ideal.

Explanation:

1. & 2. require volitional participation and a degree of discipline.

3. is semi automatic. Burning, itching, aches, pulling or drawing sensations around the eyes, cheeks, and forehead come into awareness. Practice is required to maintain this awareness.

4. is automatic. At first the breathing is slower and deeper. Later, other changes occur.

5. requires practice. When aches and pains occur, maintain awareness of them as long as possible.

6. The thinking changes from verbal to visual. Eidetic memories are experienced.

7. In some people, "releases" occur. These vary from mild twitches in muscle groups to strong jerks.

BIBLIOGRAPHY

PSYCHIATRY:
A PSYCHOPHYSIOLOGICAL SYSTEM

Baker, E.F., *Man in the Trap.* New York; Avon Books, 1974.

Bois, J.S., *The Art of Awareness.* Second edition, Dubuque, Iowa; Wm. C Brown Co., 1973.

Bonaparte, M., *Female Sexuality.* International Universities Press, Inc. New York: 1973.

Bull, N., *The Body and It's Mind.* New York; Las Americas Publishing Co., 1962.

Bull, N., The Olfactory Drive in Dislike. *Journal of Psych*ology 17:3, 1944.

Burrow, T., *Preconscious Foundations of Human Experience.* NY: Basic Books, Inc., 1964.

Burrow, T., *Science and Man's Behavior.* New York, Greenwood Press, 1968.

Chang, G.C.C., *The Practice of Zen.* New York; Perennial Library, Harper & Row, 1959.

Darwin, C., *The Expression of the Emotions in Man and Animals.* Chicago: The University of Chicago Press, 1965.

Eliade, M., *Shamanism.* New Jersey; Princeton Univ. Press, 1974.

Ellenberger, H.F., *The Discovery of the Unconscious.* New York; Basic Books, 1970.

Fischer, R., On Separateness and Oneness; *Confin. Psychiat.* 15:165, 1972.

Groddeck, G., *The Book of the It.* New York; International Universities Press, Inc., 1978.

Groddeck, G.: *The Meaning of Illness.* New York; International Universities Press, Inc., 1977.

Haley, J., *Strategies of Psychotherapy*. New York; Grune and Stratton, 1963.

Kapleau, P., *The Three Pillars of Zen*. Boston; Beacon Press, 1971.

Koryzbski, A., *Science and Sanity*. Fourth edition, Lakeville, Conn.; Non-Aristotelian Library Publishing Co. 1958.

Leary, T., *Interpersonal Diagnosis of Personality*. New York; The Roland Press, 1957.

MacLean, P.D., A Triune Concept of the Brain and Behavior in Boaq, J.J., and Campbell, D: *The Clarence M. Hincks Memorial Lecture, 1969*. Toronto; University of Toronto Press 1973.

Maier, N.R.F., *Frustration*. New York; MaGraw-Hill Book Co. 1949.

Miller, J.G., Living Systems: Basic Concepts. *Behavioral Science*, Vol. 10:3, pp. 193-37, July 1965.

Living Systems: Structure and Process. *Behavioral Science*, Vol. 10:4: 337-79 Oct.1965.

Living Systems: Cross Level Hypothesis. *Behavioral Science*, Vol. 10:4, 380-411, Oct. 1965.

Reich, W., *Character Analysis*. Third Edition, New York; The Noonday Press, 1969.

Rosett, J., The Mechanism and the Fundamental Cause of the Epilepsies. *Archives Neuro. and Psychiatry* 9:689. 1923.

Pottenger, F.M., *Symptoms of Visceral Disease, 5th edition*, St. Louis; The CV. Mosby Company, 1938.

The Books of Matthew and Job: *The Bible*. Any edition.

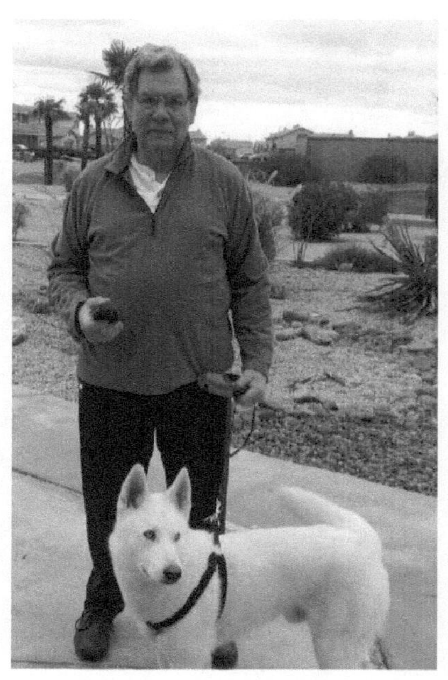

About the Author

Dr. Curtis Adams has practiced psychiatry for over forty years. At the Philadelphia Child Guidance Clinic, he trained with Jay Haley in family systems therapy. At this time, he began to develop alternative views and ways to treat the psychotic process. Dr. Adams has practiced psychiatry in various states including Alabama, Idaho and Texas. In Texas he was active in advancing protections for persons undergoing ECT treatments. Dr. Adams is now dedicating himself to writing short stories and a larger synthesis of his ideas and practice.